Chakra Meditation

The Ultimate Starter Guide to Improve Your Health and Positive Energy Learning about Chakra Meditation, and Practical Exercises to Balance and Heal Your Chakras

Sunny Heal

Table of Contents

INTRODUCTION 3

CHAPTER 1: THE BASICS OF CHAKRAS 7

    MAJOR BELIEFS OF BUDDHISM 16

CHAPTER 2: THE MAGIC OF MEDITATION 31

CHAPTER 3: TYPES OF MEDITATION 39

    TYPES OF MEDITATION 40

    BENEFITS OF MEDITATION 49

    MORNING MEDITATION 56

    NIGHT-TIME MEDITATION 57

CHAPTER 4: MEDITATION AND CHAKRAS 67

CHAPTER 5: CHAKRA MEDITATION FOR BEGINNERS 79

    BREATHING EXERCISES 85

    MINDFULNESS EXERCISES 89

CHAPTER 8: CLOSING THOUGHTS FOR YOU 102

CONCLUSION 110

Introduction

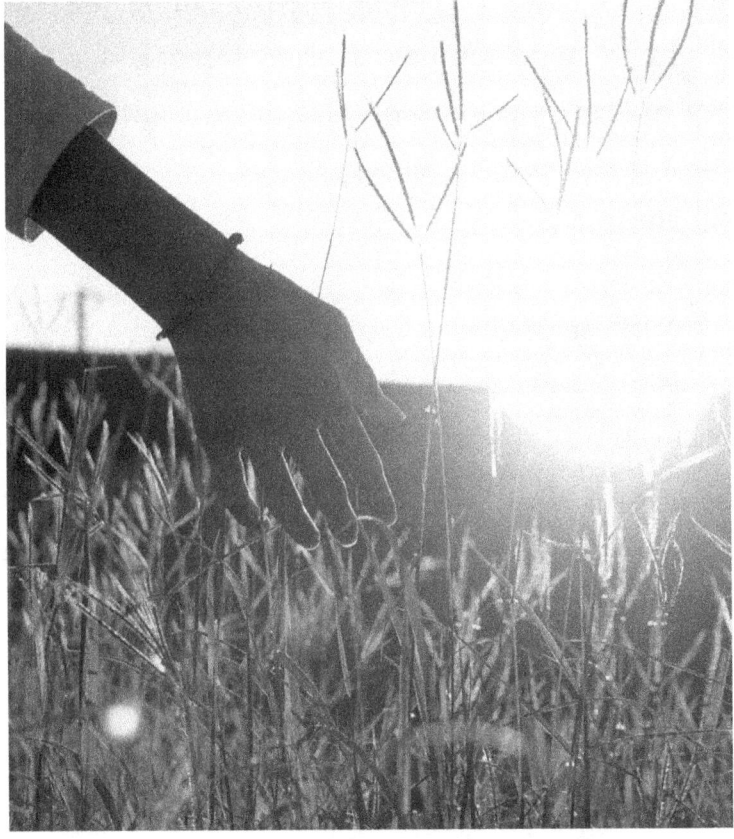

Congratulations on purchasing Chakra Meditation and thank you for doing so.

The following chapters will discuss your spiritual awakening. It is time for enlightenment, and there is much to be gained. We are entering the dawn of a new era where all things are possible. I am going to guide you on a journey through this spiritual territory you have yet to uncover. If you are reading this, you have already started your journey on the next step to being at one with the world.

If you have been feeling stressed, isolated, and out of touch lately, this is a book meant especially for you. Too often, we neglect our spiritual roots and leave untended the garden in our minds. Opening up your chakras and letting energy flow freely to your crown is the cure for all of this and more. You will never feel more at peace with yourself than when you bring yourself back to this perfect center. The answers are in you, I am just the conduit for the experience.

From here, I will explore multiple topics which deal with Chakras. From meditation, to mindfulness and beyond, you will learn everything there is to know. Chakras are essential to opening up the energy in your body and becoming in tune with the needs of your spirit. Everything rides on the oneness inherent in the universe, and this return to self is dependent on your enlightenment.

For a taste of what is to come:
- How to practice mindfulness
- Morning rituals for peaceful days
- Bedtime meditation for restful nights
- Every form of meditation which draws on spiritual energy
- ... and much, much more

I will leave no stone left unturned in the pursuit of empowering you to move forward on this path. My goal is to inspire you so that you might be better motivated for it. There is much work to be done, and sometimes it may feel tedious, but all of these things are necessary to bringing your energy into balance.

There are plenty of books on this subject on the market, thanks again for choosing this one! Every effort was made to ensure it is full of as much useful information as possible, please enjoy!

Chapter 1: The Basics of Chakras

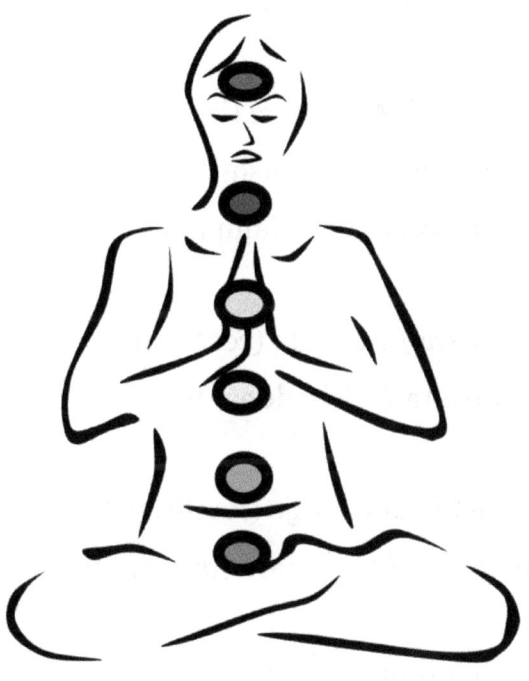

The first place to start is, of course, with chakras themselves. In this chapter, I will only go over basics, and some interesting facts and history. I just want to get your feet wet so that you have a solid foundation from which to build following this section. Chakras are multi-faceted by nature and steeped in mysticism. It takes quite a bit to explain them in full.

Have you near, however, because I am going to break it down for you. Let us get right into it!

There are a list of chakras, which I will go over below:

- Root Chakra / Muladhara (bottom of *the* spine)
- Sacral Chakra / Swaddhishthana (pelvic region)
- Solar Plexus Chakra / Manipura (naval area and slightly above)
- Heart Chakra / Anahata (center of the chest)
- Throat Chakra / Vishuddha (where *the* throat meets *the* neck)
- Third Eye Chakra / Anja (forehead, between the eyes)
- Crown Chakra / Sahasrara (the very top of your head)

This may seem like quite the list to learn, but I promise you that when I go over them in detail in a chapter further along it will all come together beautifully. Chakras line all the way up your body. Your entirety is based on these center points of spiritual power. You should use them as your compass and guide. There can be no true awakening, no true enlightenment, without having free-flowing energy. This can only be attained with clean, well-maintained chakras.

However, there is a little bit you need to know before we get into that whole cleaning business. For starters, there are other names these chakras go by. This is because of their roots in eastern philosophy. They are based on ancient words from an ancient language called Sanskrit, and it is the foundation of many languages we know today.

I would argue that this carries some serious power. There is something about the archaic nature of Sanskrit that seems to carry some sort of ancient wisdom. I truly believe that this transfers through the texts used to describe these practices. It is because Sanskrit is so old that we know practicing these rituals and meditation forms go further back than ever previously thought.

While you might view people, who practice meditation or get involved with chakras as "crunchy hippies", let it be known that this could not be further from the truth. In fact, these practices predate many religions as we know them now. The original word for chakras actually originated as far back as 1500bc. That is an insanely long time ago. I think that there is something to be said about ancient wisdom and what we can gain from it. Learning about chakras inspires a recognition of your place in the universe and peacefulness which comes with that knowledge.

To begin, for those of you who have not read my first book "Chakras for beginners", let me give you a solid definition of the word "Chakra". This should help even the most basic beginners begin to form a better idea of what this book is all about. I will go over the idea of "Prana", which is another essential word we will be using all the way to the last chapter of this book.

- **Chakra:** Comes from the Sanskrit word for "disk" or "wheel". These are the spiritual powerhouses within your body. They provide a method through which *Prana* can flow uninhibited through your body. When a chakra is blocked, you feel certain effects due to this disconnect between body, spirit, and mind.
- **Prana:** The life-force which flows through us all. This is the energy that chakras allow to pass through our body. They heal us, keep us revitalized, and inspire vibrancy within us.
- **Nirvana:** The result of enlightenment. Once you have lived your life correctly, you are allowed to enter a state of nirvana. This is what all Buddhists seek to reach as the "highest echelon" of having been spiritually awakened. You can think of it as the Buddhist version of heaven.
- **Buddha:** Some may tell you this is the "God" of Buddhism. While you may be able to draw parallels, the

Buddha is not actually a God at all. More on that below, however, when I go over some of the major beliefs of Buddhism.

- **Karma:** This is not the idea of your fate which has been predetermined. Many in the public arena seem to think this, but it is largely untrue. Instead, karma explains the positive and negative actions of a person through their life journey.

  Each action you have carries a certain weight and contributes to your happiness in the long run.

Remember these! In fact, it may be a good idea to bookmark this page so you can come back to it if you need a refresher on these words. Having so much new terminology and information thrown at you can be highly overwhelming. I am going to try and get it boiled down enough that you will not have too much trouble.

You may be wondering how chakras came about, and what their history is. I think it is only fair to go over this part more in-depth so that you can understand the rich, far-extending history that goes behind these practices that lay ahead.

Chakras come from ancient eastern philosophy. They originated in India, somewhere between 1500 BCE and 500 BCE within the Hindu Vedas. These are a large body of religious texts composed in Vedic Sanskrit. They did not originally appear with the term Chakras and in the sense of mystical energy, thus the exact time of origin cannot be calculated. However, the best evidence suggests that this really is one of the most ancient practices out there.

Things that have been around for over a thousand years are engrained into our evolution. This is true of many things. Chakras are simply a natural progression born from the understanding which our ancient ancestors had. It is much like understanding our role as small parts of the whole- that is, after all, what this is all about. The idea of chakras was passed down through oral tradition, or, more simply put, by word of mouth. This is another reason tracking down the earliest mention of chakras so difficult. You can find references to chakras in the following texts:

- *Shri Jabala Darshana Upanishad*
- *Cudamini Upanishad*
- *Yoga-Shikka Upanishad*
- *Shandilya Upanishad*

While this has become considered a "new-age" belief, this is a white-washing of the traditions. Again, it originated in eastern philosophy. There were parts of Europe that began to be influenced by this. However, with the rise of Christianity and the fall of polytheism, the idea of chakras was chased quickly out of other parts of the world. It held its ground and stayed in common understanding in India, however, and the surrounding countries.

We have to be thankful for some of the scholars and researchers who brought this practice back into the popular eye, however. It is because of them that many of us are able to partake in the cleansing of our chakras and come back to being one with ourselves as well as the universe around us. Enlightenment is possible, and especially through the careful cleansing of your energy channels.

You can imagine a chakra in this way: a constantly spinning "wheel" of energy which allows for the free flow of *Prana*, our life force. What you may not know is that there are many more chakra centers throughout the body. In fact, some believe there are as many as 114. However, because this is a book for beginners, I am going to stick to those seven chakras which are so prominent and important.

Chakras are not just influenced by *Prana*, however. There is much more which goes into them. The cleansing of your chakras is comprised of three different methods:

- **Physical:** Your body is your vessel. This is the place in which you reside for the time being. Whether your physical body is in good standing or not relies heavily on your daily activities. You need to ensure you are getting the correct amount of exercise, as well as eating a diet that nurtures you. It is popular to eat a plant-based diet among many people who practice Buddhism or Hinduism.

   However, a plant-based diet is, obviously, not a requirement. It is just a consideration you should make for the overall health of your body.

- **Mental:** There are multiple illnesses that require medication. I am not in the least advocating for people to go off these medications. Instead, I simply want to highlight the positive impact which cleansing your chakras has on your mental health. They are intrinsically connected since a clear mind helps chakras stay squeaky clean, and clean chakras help your mind stay clear.

Mental health is, perhaps, the most important component for your immediate attention.

- **Spiritual:** Of course, I have to talk about the spiritual energy growing within you. With each word, I hope you will become more in tune with it! Your spiritual health is dictated mostly by you. You need to do what you feel is best to nurture that growth. Engaging in the exercises and guided meditations I will give to you in later chapters is a great start, however.

It is important to remember that you must take care of your entirety. You cannot hope to accomplish a true cleansing until you begin to see your entire body as a system. All things are interconnected, which is the exact lesson that I am looking to teach you.

References to chakras are now found commonly. You can walk into almost any "hippie" or new-age shop and find all of the stones, incense, and other supplies you need for properly done meditation or other spiritual practices.

Let us talk a little bit more about Buddhism. This is, after all, the religion that focuses the most on *Prana* and the cleansing of chakras. It is an essential part of their belief systems. I am going to run down a list of Buddhist beliefs and considerations.

Major Beliefs of Buddhism

- **There is no supreme being that they worship.** This is probably one of the healthiest aspects of this religion. Your aim is not to worship a God. Instead, your aim is to practice strong morality and achieve enlightenment.
- **Buddha was not a God, but simply an enlightened man.** Many people get this part wrong. If you ask somebody off the streets who Buddhists worship, they might give you Buddha as an answer. However, as mentioned, there are no Gods in this religion. In fact, his very name, Buddha, actually means "enlightened".

    As a fun piece of trivia, originally the Buddha's name was Siddhartha Gautama.
- **It is based on strong morality.** There is no life too small to respect in a Buddhist's eyes. These peaceful people prefer to focus on cultivating their wisdom and keeping their mind open to spiritual awakening. This is

why such a strong focus on cleansing chakras and meditation is held by many.

- **Buddhism branches off in several directions.** As I had mentioned prior in this list, this is an ever-evolving religion (or philosophy, depending on who you ask). There are multiple circles and styles of practice which you can explore. This is another reason why Buddhism resonates with so many. Because of the options available, you can always find a way to practice which fits perfectly for you.

- **Some are of the opinion that Buddhism is not a true "religion".** Generally speaking, it is scholars who hold this. Because of the lack of components, you see in mainstream religions, such as the lack of a God or supreme being, some argue it just does not qualify. However, most practicing Buddhists would readily argue this.

- **It borrows concepts from other philosophies and religions.** Because of this, it is consistently and constantly morphing. Buddhism tends to err on the side of acceptance and tolerance. Many scholars believe that this is because of the evolving nature of this philosophy.

- **Their code of conduct is based on the "The Four Noble Truths".** I will go over these more below and tell you what they are. Essentially, they are the Buddhist version of the 10 Commandments which Christians live by.

These are beliefs that many people can get behind. The surge to join Buddhism gets stronger and stronger as we move into a culture drenched in the pursuit of mindfulness. This is one of the best things that the age of this era brought to us. The spread of eastern philosophies in the western world has led us down a path to better enlightenment as a society. It is my hope that helping you through all of this information will help you do the same! After all, we are simply parts of a whole. By doing your part as a practicing Buddhist, or somebody who simply follows the philosophies, you are doing your part in cleansing the chakras of the world. Metaphorically speaking, of course.

Now, onto the last bit of basics concerning Buddhism that I think you need to know immediately. These are The Four Noble Truths which I mentioned earlier. They are the most sacred and important teachings passed down by Buddha himself. You are to follow these at all times on your pursuit of Nirvana.

The Buddha's life story is meant to serve as an example of how every person should live their life. If you follow in his footsteps, you will be well on your way to the enlightenment promised to you.

Below you will find the main tenants you must follow as a Buddhist, whether practicing it as a religion or as a general philosophy to guide you through life. While they may seem simplistic at first, you need to recognize the profoundness of Buddha's teachings. At the time, these were revolutionary ideas unfounded largely in the rest of the world. They were far, far ahead of the curve. There are actually things the Buddha alluded to that had not even come to light yet. More on that later, however, as we begin to explore these topics further. Without further delay, here are those Four Noble Rules of Buddhism I have been promising.

The Four Noble Rules of Buddhism:

- **The Truth of Suffering (Dukkha):** The idea that our will have suffering we cannot avoid. It is entirely inevitable. There are several different ways in which this is shown to be true. Chronic illness, as well as loss and the grief which follows, are great examples of this first rule.

Here are some examples of physical suffering:
- Arthritis
- Headaches
- Cramps
- General illness

Here are some examples of mental suffering:
- Disappointment
- Heartache
- Depression
- Anxiety

This first rule encompasses a simple truth about the world that we all understand, even on merely a subconscious level.

- **The Truth of the Cause of Suffering (Samudaya or Tanha):** Simply put, this is your attachment to your desire. Craving of any sort, whether for physical comforts or materialistic gain, falls into this category. It is the Buddha's belief that you must let go of everything you want in order to gain true enlightenment. Desire is the opponent of enlightenment. It causes us to be unhappy with what we have in the current moment. Being at peace with yourself and allowing the free flow of *Prana* to run through your body is essential. Holding on to the things you lust over, and that lust, is the cause of your despair and dysregulation of energy.

- **The Truth of the End of Suffering (Nirodha):** When you are able to let go of these desires and lustful thoughts, you can achieve true enlightenment. What ends this suffering is letting go. You must be able to embody the idea of dispassion. In order to achieve Nirvana, you must stay mindful and at peace with what you have. Those who have not yet begun living the rule of Nirodha will not be able to achieve Nirvana. They have not yet achieved freedom from their worries, troublesome ideas, and different desires. This is a key factor in earning your place in the state of Nirvana.

- **The Truth of the Path that Leads to the End of Suffering (Eightfold Path):** Now, that is quite the title! However, I am sure you can see how the natural progression led us here. I will also go over the Eightfold Path, but for now just know that this is how you achieve freedom from suffering. Not many people will reach this level. Only those who are truly enlightened can hope to free themselves of suffering.

I think I will leave you here on the topic of Buddhism. This was a short introduction, but you will be building off of it from here on out. For now, simply remember to follow those four rules closely in your day-to-day life. This is not simply a matter of practicing Buddhism, either. These moral codes are meant to bring you closer to enlightenment. Making sure your energy channels are clear and working correctly means bringing yourself closer to Nirvana as a general rule.

As promised, I will quickly list out the Eightfold Path. This is fairly self-explanatory, so I do not think I need to flesh out what, exactly, they are.

- Right view
- Right effort
- Right concentration
- Right livelihood
- Right speech
- Right intention
- Right action
- Right mindfulness

Ensuring that you are going down this path and practicing the Four Noble Rules of Buddhism is the slow, arduous path one must take to reach Nirvana.

Now, let us talk about how chakras come into play in everyday life. This will be a nice way to round out this chapter so that we can focus on our next topic, meditation. Get excited because you are going to be chock-full of ways to meditate every single day. For now, however, let us focus on those daily uses of chakras and how they come into play during your everyday life.

Each of the chakras has a different focus relating to your physical and mental wellbeing. The strategic points at which they are placed translate to a deep understanding of the way the body works. I am going to go ahead and list out those chakras again, and put down what, exactly, they focus on the most. This will be your first introduction to the power chakras wield in your everyday life. As we progress through the book, I will lay out more and more on the topic.

Crown Chakra
This is the chakra that lays at the very top of your head. When you stretch upwards to encourage energy flow, you are focusing things upwards towards your crown. Here are some of the ways in which it is used every day:

- Your overall connection to the world around you is affected by the crown chakra.

- Crown chakra is also responsible for connecting you to ecstasy and bringing you closer to Nirvana.
- Union with the all-mighty flow of *Prana*, or life energy, is dictated by the crown chakra.

Third Eye Chakra

Probably one of the most popularized chakras, the third eye means so much more than just some tired, old saying or trope. This is the most important chakra for making your daily decisions. Some places where you will activate it throughout your daily routine are as follows:

- Vision is deeply affected by the third eye chakra. However, I do not mean this in the traditional sense. I mean your vision regarding all things, whether spiritual or physical.
- Third eye chakra also has a hand in building yourself up intellectually. This means finding the truth of things and understanding concepts as they are presented.

Throat Chakra

If you are having trouble with interpersonal relationships, you are in desperate need of clearing your throat chakra. This is so incredibly important... and especially so for anybody who works with people daily! All of your important relationships ride on the free flow of *Prana* through this source.

- If you have ever heard the term "powerhouse", then you already know quite a bit about the throat chakra. This is the place from which your true power with people comes from.
- The ability to have strong leadership skills is closely related to the throat chakra. This is especially important for leaders to clear and regulate.

Heart Chakra

Ensuring that you are living a life that causes as little suffering to others as possible is tantamount to reaching the state of Nirvana. The heart chakra is here to help you do just that. There are many places in your life where this will come into play daily. Here are just a few of those ways:

- Ultimately, your goal for Buddhism is to find love in yourself for all beings. The heart chakra allows for more compassionate living in your day to day life.

- The heart chakra is also necessary for having a strong sense of inner peace. Love is connected to this- if you cannot find inner peace, it will be hard to find love for all the beings around you.

Solar Plexus Chakra

One punch, and you are done! All jokes aside, this is actually true of the chakra which controls both the emotions and digestion. These are two critical parts of your life! Both are inwardly directed but the state of this chakra will highly control your interactions with others. And, of course, yourself. Below you will find the ways in which this is experienced daily:

- Your emotions are a huge part of your ability to be healthy in your entirety. In your everyday life, this is the chakra holds power over your emotions. Keep it clean and clear in order to have better success in your emotional regulation.
- Of course, digestion is also a big part of this chakra. That plays into the idea I presented earlier. This idea, of course, is that you must be healthy physically, mentally, and spiritually to reach true enlightenment.

Sacral Chakra

If you remember the Four Noble Rules of Buddhism, this chakra will make a whole lot of sense. It is connected to two things: pleasure, and your well-being materialistically. This encompasses more about your ability to have shelter, food, and other daily necessities, rather than the material things you may be used to thinking of. Of course, now that we live in a world where material things are tantamount to the image of success, it has become morphing to mean that, as well.

Here are those situations you will face where it will come highly into play:

- Those day-to-day pleasures you engage in are connected to your Sacral chakra. This is where your pleasure comes from- both literally and figuratively.
- Depression can, in part, be treated by the regular clearing of this chakra.

Root Chakra

Finally, we have the last chakra along your spine. This is the root chakra which has full control over both your security, as well as your instincts.

Clearing the root chakra is the first step in making sure all of your channels are clear. This is your base from which all other things must grow. Your root chakra being clear will help you in the following ways:

- This is the first chakra which you will be clearing. It is the root of everything- your basic need for survival. Root chakra keys in to your overall security as well as your instinct-driven behaviors.

Now that you have what you need for a solid foundation, I think it is time to round off this chapter. Hopefully it managed to convey a few ideas and educate you on the ideas surrounding Buddhism, chakras, and a few more topics you need. It is always a good idea to use this chapter as reference through the rest of the books. From here out, I will be using the terms described freely and liberally. Ensure that you know what they are so things can be communicated more clearly for you.

Now we will move on to one of the most practical chapters in the book. Next we are going to talk all about meditation! Expect guided exercises, different forms to use, and so much more.

Chapter 2: The Magic of Meditation

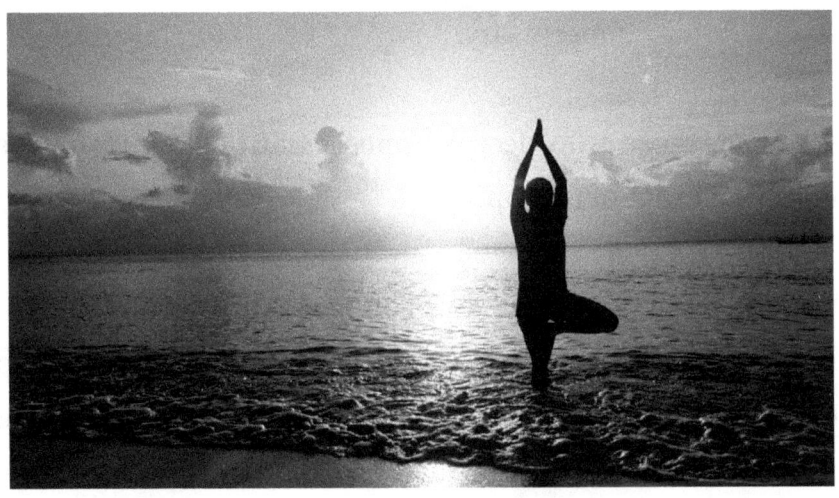

The Rich History, the Overall Mindset and More

Ah, yes! This chapter is going to be one I am sure you are excited to read. But not nearly as excited as I am to write it! I love giving practical exercises and examples for you so that you can further your education in a more realistic way. After all, I can tell you all about meditation and chakras until I am blue in the face (or fingers). That does nothing to help you move forward towards serenity and enlightenment, however.

So, what is meditation, exactly? I know that you must have heard of it. This is a highly popularized activity that most people have a very strong opinion on. It is seen as tedious at best and, at worst, totally unnecessary.

Of course, those who deem it unnecessary or unhelpful are entirely ignorant of the topic.

I want to give you a full rundown on meditation here. This, just like in the previous chapter, will give you the base you need to build off. I am going to go over the general history, including the geographical origin of meditation. On top of this, I will give you multiple types of meditation you can practice and the benefits of them.

The type of meditation we are going to explore was originally developed in India. I am sure there is no surprise there since that seems to be the origin point for most topics in this book. There are many pieces of ancient wall art that show the use of meditation being used as far back as 5,000 BCE. This shows that meditation grew and formed at least simultaneously to Buddhism. The truth is, however, that the two probably share the same origin and simply split as time moved forward.

The practice of meditation can be seen all over the globe. However, we cannot forget its roots in eastern philosophy- more specifically, India.

It is not just Buddhists who took to the idea of meditation, however. You will see many other eastern philosophies and religions drawing from the power offered by meditation. Taoism, which is a religion originating in China, is a prime example of this. Each of these eastern philosophies has generally developed its own form of meditation or several different forms. The best part about meditation is that there are so many different types out there that it makes it easy to find one you truly mesh with.

Do not be mistaken, however. There is definitely scholarly proof that meditation also took hold in the west. This is mainly due to the obvious power inherent in meditative practices. Practicing mindfulness is one of the best ways to encourage your overall happiness and feelings of internal serenity.

The word meditation actually comes from the French word *"meditacioun"*, rather than Sanskrit. This, in turn, comes from the Latin word *"meditatio"*, which translates roughly to "to think or reflect upon".

However, the Buddha was, of course, a huge proponent of meditation. In fact, this is one of the practices that brings you to a state of enlightenment. This is why clearing your chakras through meditation is crucial for your path to inner, and outer peace. Making sure that you understand the world around you as it truly is will also play a crucial role, and is another area in which meditation, and mindfulness, help you. As you can imagine, conducting yourself in an ethical manner is the last of these three.

There are several uses for meditation, and the benefits are too many to name. I will do my best to make sure you understand almost every benefit there is, nonetheless, I want you to have a full comprehension of the power that meditation can provide. Cleaning your chakras properly requires the usage of meditation… and the proper usage, at that. Have no fear on that end, however. I will be going over everything you need in the way of exercises.

First, let me go over the major benefits you can gain from daily meditation.

- **Enhancing self-awareness:** The path to enlightenment begins with self-reflection or spending some time at peace with the world. As you begin to explore the inner realms of yourself, you will begin to cultivate self-awareness. This is something everybody could stand to gain. There is a growing problem with a lack of self-awareness, mainly due to the modern technology available.

Spending some time away from everything locked in a meditative state will always bring you a better overall awareness.

- **Generate external kindness:** Making sure you do right by others is not just a constituent of Buddhism. It is also a tenant of constituent human decency. Participating in daily meditation is proven to help people practice kindness towards others. There is something about the inner peace that pushes you to provide others with the same peace of mind.
- **Regulates emotional health:** When you feel as though your emotions are out of control, turning to meditation can be a healthy way to deal with it. Regulating your emotions will come easier and easier as you explore the depths of meditation. Emotional balance is the cornerstone of inner peace and a better life overall.
- **Grants better concentration:** If you have trouble with concentration, meditation has an answer for that. It

has been shown scientifically that experiencing the clarity that meditation is so known for will often bring you better concentration overall. It tells your brain to slow down and think more rationally about things.

- **Builds mental connections:** Speaking of which, meditation has also been shown to help build new connections in the brain. Since you are entering a state of mindfulness, it is almost like being "asleep" while you are awake. When you sleep, you are building connections in your brain. You can trick your brain into thinking you are sleeping by slowing down your body and entering true mindfulness.

- **Keeps anxiety levels low:** This goes hand in hand with the idea of emotional regulation. Even beyond this, however, is the pursuit of lowering anxiety levels. For some, this is a serious disorder that requires treatment. Most therapists will strongly suggest picking up mindfulness or meditation to help cope.

In fact, it is a crucial part of one of the most popular, and successful, treatment methods currently available. This treatment is called "Cognitive Behavioral Therapy" if you were curious!

- **Allows for better stress management:** Overall stress is a huge contributor to people being unhappy and overwhelmed. Bringing your stress levels down is crucial to living a happy, full life. Meditation gives you the opportunity to put your worries, fears, and anger aside for a few minutes. This gives you the chance to cool down and think about things more rationally afterward.

Remember that the list of benefits is exhaustive and could go on forever. These are just a few of the ways I think meditation benefits common people in their day-to-day lives. You will also notice that while we talk about meditation I will step further away from Buddhism on the whole. While this is a crucial thing to understand on your road to understanding chakras, I want it to be also appealing to anybody who may be reading this.

The truth is that you do not have to practice Buddhism to meditate or practice mindfulness. You will be doing so on "accident", but consciously doing so is not necessarily required.

Chapter 3: Types of Meditation

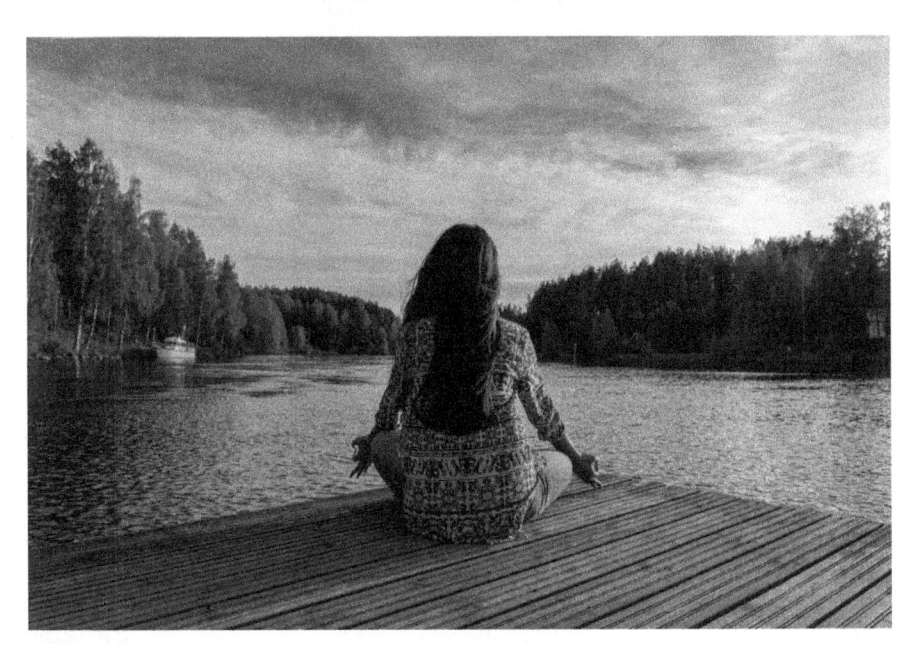

Everything on the Different Forms of Meditation

Now that I have gone over the benefits and general history of meditation, let me move right into the meat of the matter. I think it is high time to talk about the different forms of meditation you can engage with. This should give you a selection of practices, which you can easily choose from.

I want to ensure that every person who reads this book will walk away with a form of meditation that they can enjoy practicing. I will not be going over guided meditation quite yet- instead, I want you to focus on understanding these four types of meditation. Hone in on which ones feel "right" to you, and which you think would be best for your particular situation.

Types of Meditation

Spiritual Meditation

Remember earlier when I said you do not necessarily have to be a Buddhist to gain the benefits of meditation? Most people associate meditation with eastern religions and philosophies- and rightly so! However, there are actually many Judeo-Christian religions that practice the art of meditation.

While clearing your chakras is necessary no matter which religion you prescribe to, I want to make sure that everybody reading this knows that it is not contradictory to their beliefs.

The best part about non-theistic philosophies, such as Buddhism and Taoism, is that they encourage you to become a better human being. That is the main goal. There is no underlying intention or need to convert others. The goal is to simply be better, more understanding, and encourage the growth of self-awareness.

Meditation can be utilized as a way to feel closer to your current religion. You can practice this form at your place of worship, or just at your house. It is a great way to make sure your *Prana* is flowing freely, and your energy is aligned, alongside bringing you closer to your faith.

The benefits of this meditation are as follows:
- **A stronger relationship with your higher power.** If you practice any religion, you know how important the relationship with your chosen deity is. We look to our God(s) for comfort, strength, and the answers we search for. Meditation is one of the best ways to bring yourself to a state of mindfulness and feel the power of your belief system rolling through you.
- **The cultivation of inner peace.** One of the biggest aims of religion is to give us the feeling of peace that helps us live in harmony with the world around us.

Meditation, at its core, is about bettering yourself and growing internally. Combining this with your spiritual and religious beliefs is a sure-fire way to gain the benefits of both- and so, so much more.

- **There is more wiggle room as far as religious beliefs go.** While I will be pushing Buddhism, both as a philosophy and a religion, I understand that it may not be what you believe. I do not want you to think that these practices are reserved for a certain "type" of the person with a limited belief system attached. Instead, know that there are ways to incorporate the teachings of the Buddha into any religion you practice. You can look at this as a philosophy you are bringing into your life.

Mindfulness Meditation

These are two words I have used repeatedly thus far! However, you will find that they are the two most powerful practices you can bring into your life. Mindfulness is a fantastic way to bring yourself back to the center, improve your emotional health, clear your mind, and more. I will talk far more about mindfulness later on in the book. I will also, of course, be going over quite a few guided meditations in relation to this particular style of both mindfulness and meditation.

There are a few goals of mindfulness, but in general, the main goal is to cultivate awareness within yourself. It serves as the base from which you will begin to build the tools to overcome stress, impatience, intolerance, and more. These are all things we could stand to lessen in the world. Mindfulness meditation is a great way to do that.

The benefits of this meditation are as follows:

- **It is a great regulator for emotions.** Many people struggle with anxiety and stress, especially in this new age of constant access to others and digital disorder. Making sure that your emotions are regulated is an important part of staying healthy mentally. Building yourself up against this hectic world and the extra stressors it brings is paramount to your success.
- **Mindfulness is scientifically proven to help treat disorders.** Notice how I did not specify physical or mental? As it turns out, mindfulness helps both. There are several studies showing the positive effects that mindfulness has on those who practice it. Chronic pain stands to gain quite a bit from meditating in this style. The same goes for all mental illnesses. Again, the most popular treatment style, Cognitive Behavioral Therapy, draws deeply from the well of mindfulness.

- **Those who practice mindfulness are shown to live happier, healthier lives.** The overall happiness and peace you feel will increase exponentially when you invite mindfulness into your life. Most of us are caught up with our day-to-day worries, stressed about things that have happened... or those things that only may happen. Mindfulness reminds us to live in the current moment and to put away the fears that haunt our thoughts.

Movement Meditation

For those of you who may not enjoy sitting still, this is the perfect answer. Movement meditation is the answer for those who are filled with too much energy to stay in one place for too long. There are several different avenues you can go down in order to use this form of meditation. In fact, I would greatly encourage you to explore how it can be used specifically for you. The best part about movement meditation is that it tends to fit better into our lives.

For example, if you enjoy working out, you can begin to incorporate this meditation into your stretching and cool-down period. The point of meditation, especially in reference to active movement meditation, is to have the ability to incorporate it easily into your life.

There are many, many ways in which to incorporate this particular form of meditation into your daily life. I want to make sure you find the exact correct form for you so that cleansing your energy and aligning yourself will be a breeze.

As it turns out, movement meditation tends to be the answer for many!

The benefits of this meditation are as follows:

- **Meditation happens on your schedule, no matter what.** It is much easier to engage with meditation when you do not have to clear a specific time of your day for it. Movement meditation is fantastic because you can incorporate it into almost anything that you do. While mindfulness is another form that can be used in such a way, movement meditation is a specific off-shoot. It uses your active body in such a way that *Prana* is able to flow freely and actively.
- **You can engage with movement meditation at any time.** Being in the practice of movement meditation is a fantastic way to slowly dip your toes into the water, so to speak. It does not require anything special or fancy. You will not be required to set up a special space. You can dive right in and bring it with you

everywhere you go. This is the best place to start if you are still feeling unsure about meditation.
- **There are many benefits to stretching and moving.** Your body will thank you for putting more effort into regular exercise. Most people think of running or lifting weights when they think of exercise, but this is not the case. Something as simple as getting up from your desk and running through some deep stretches can be extremely beneficial. Your cardiovascular system will thank you! Incorporating meditation into it takes it another step in the right direction to better health and a happier life.

Visualization Meditation

This is perhaps one of the best forms of meditation to engage in if you are planning for future goals. Visualization is used in a variety of cultures and ways to "manifest" things toward you. The idea of manifestation has been passed down for thousands of years and shows up in almost every single ancient religion, but especially those polytheistic ones, which fell out of favor. Visualization is also a form of mindfulness!

In some cultures, this is a religious practice. Most notably, we can look at the Tibetan monks, who use it as a form of cultivating better wisdom, faith, and higher levels of compassion.

When you engage in visualization meditation, you are going to be doing just that- visualizing. There is no one right way to do it, but I will give you a bunch of exercises in a chapter coming soon so you know where to start. Most of the time you are going to be envisioning a triumph, or something you want. More on that later, however!

The benefits of this meditation are as follows:
- **Visualization allows for a surge of positivity in your life.** You will absolutely find, as you begin to practice, that you are more at peace with the state of things. Oftentimes we are unhappy because we are constantly trying to figure out how to get the next best "thing". Whether this is a material object or a station in life, most of us are doggedly obsessed with moving "up" in the world. Visualization allows you to be more at peace with what you have, and more confident in the growth towards what you want.
- **Imagining your success is a great way to manifest it.** Again, there is a lot of science backing this up. More and more we are seeing that visualization and manifestation are highly positive activities for the brain to participate in. Even if you do not actually "will" something toward you, you are certainly setting yourself up for success mentally. Being confident is a huge part of

moving forward in life, and visualization will help you cultivate that confidence.

- **On the other hand, this provides a great way to be at peace with not getting what you want.** At the end of the day, we cannot always get what we want (not quoting the Rolling Stones here). We must be happy and content with the things we currently have. If you remember the main attributes of Buddhism, then you remember that this is one of the goals. Letting go of desire and want is the goal for those seeking Nirvana.

I think that should be enough for now. These are four common types of meditation that have been largely proven to help the vast majority of people who practice them. The "correct" form of meditation, however, is the one that you are able to do daily. Always remember that things can look great on paper. If you are not using them, though, they do nothing for you. Make sure you are going with a form of meditation that speaks to you personally and you think will be doable in your daily life. The goal is not to change your life to fit meditation- the goal is to choose the meditation that fits your life. This will produce far better results and make it vastly easier for you to stick with.

I think that I have gone over quite a bit in the way of forms of meditation. There will be more I go over later, make no mistake, but for now, let us move into the main benefits of meditation. I will also be going over how using chakras in a daily setting can benefit you.

There are several benefits to using meditation daily, as well as having clear chakras. I am going to go down a quick list of some examples where most people need better management. I think after reading this list, you will have a much better understanding of where exactly, meditation can benefit you.

I will not go too deeply into these benefits. I went through some earlier, so for now here are some more quick and simple ones. I will separate these between mental, physical, and emotional benefits.

Benefits of Meditation

Mental Benefits
- Improves your focus
- Allows for better creative thinking
- Manages multiple different mental illnesses
- Helps you filter out distractions
- Encourages the development of good memory

- Gives you better information recall
- Increases overall creativity in thinking

Emotional Benefits

- Controls anxiety and worry
- Helps curb impulsive behavior
- Heightens resilience against adversity
- Allows for better interpersonal communication
- Teaches better emotional intelligence
- Improves overall mood

Physical Benefits

- Evens out heart rate
- Lowers resting heart rate
- Increases longevity of life
- Counters the effects of arthritis
- Minimizes pain from Fibromyalgia
- Keeps blood pressure low
- Improves cardiovascular health

That is quite the laundry list of benefits! I am sure at this point that you have a much better understanding of why meditation is so important to your everyday life. It has been shown repeatedly that those who incorporate meditation into their daily lives are going to be happier, healthier, and more resilient. The key to life is perseverance, and meditation helps you cultivate this all too necessary skill.

However, that is only half the battle. There are even more benefits I promised to go over, and now it is time to move into the subject at hand: chakras. While meditation is fantastic on its own, you should always be focusing on those energy centers within your body. Cleansing them and realigning yourself is crucial for your continued happiness and ability to move through life freely.

I mentioned earlier how there are more than 7 chakras in the body. For now, however, we will only focus on those main 7 that are so popularized today. Once you begin to delve deeper into this subject you will move forward in your knowledge. Most people do not study or use the other chakras unless they are dedicated to yogis or practicing Buddhists. Getting you started out with knowledge on the first 7 chakras is going to get you off to the start you need.

We will go over the benefits of each, one by one. I will, of course, be going far deeper into the chakras in the next chapter. That is where I will be marrying all of this information and where everything will make perfect sense. For now, I want to get you set-up for that by giving you a taste of what is to come.

Root Chakra Benefits
- Helps harness confidence in the most basic sense
- Encourages grounding and stability
- Allows for you to "root" yourself into reality
- Reminds us of our humble origins
- Keeps us feeling stable

Sacral Chakra
- Controls feelings of pleasure
- Encourages you to act selflessly
- Creates a stronger connection to the world
- Allows for the cultivation of intuition
- Helps curb negative emotions such as loneliness or depression
- Enhances your ability to be insightful

Solar Plexus Chakra
- Encourages the development of self-control
- Can help boost your confidence

- Keeps us feeling level and secure
- Helps lower feelings of insecurity

Heart Chakra

- Fills us with self-love and acceptance
- Allows for a better understanding of others
- Increases the love we pour out into the world
- Brings feelings of joy to you
- Regulates blood pressure
- Brings heartbeat back into the rhythm
- Encourages feelings of inner-peace

Throat Chakra

- Improves communication with others
- Balances interpersonal relationships
- Helps us "hear" what others are saying
- Motivates us to release negative thought patterns
- Brings peace in the face of weakness or fear
- Encourages better self-expression internally and externally

Third Eye Chakra

- Soothes our fears of the unknown
- Counters stressors of everyday life

- Reminds us of our small place in this large world
- Encourages us to remember the "bigger picture"
- Helps us cultivate wisdom
- Allows for better intuition to develop

Crown Chakra
- Encourages better spiritual connection with the self
- Also encourages spiritual connection to the world
- The main gateway through which *Prana* enters
- Feelings of ecstasy are largely felt through this chakra
- Builds connections to either spirituality or chosen deity

As you can see, there are many, many benefits to each chakra being used daily. The cleansing of these energy centers is a crucial part of living the healthiest life you can. True enlightenment and oneness are possible for all beings. We cannot control that we are part of this world. We can only control how much we value our place in it. Understanding your chakras, keeping them clean and engaging in meditation allows for a happier, longer, more fulfilled life.

I have talked quite a bit about how important meditation is in your daily life. How do you set up the right space, however? And when should you practice? That is exactly what this section is going to cover before we move more into the links between chakras and meditation specifically. Having the correct space in which to practice is tantamount to your success. You cannot hope to be in the right mindset if you do not have the right space in which to do so. There are a few ways in which you can maximize the return you get on this "investment"; that is, the investment you are putting into your life through cleansing your chakras.

Normally, you want to put yourself into a comfortable routine. There is a lot to be gained when you commit to a routine, after all. We need to make sure our brains and bodies know that we are going to engage in this form of spiritual exercise. When you meditate on a regular schedule daily, you will begin to feel the full effects far more quickly than if, you do it at random. Schedules are important to all aspects of life, but especially in the pursuit of self-improvement.

I recommend tackling this in one of two ways. You can either do so in the morning or at night. The point is to set yourself up for a day of inner peace and acceptance or to slow down your body and brain at night for better sleep.

Morning Meditation

The meditation, which you do in the morning, should engage the chakras, which will help you, find peace throughout your day. The meditation style should energize you, bring you inner peace, and hone your mind for the activities to follow. You can practice any of the forms of meditation you would like. However, I suggest the meditation exercises below.

- **Personal Mantra Meditation:** The first step in a bountiful day full of confidence and blessings is, to begin with, your personal mantras. This is not a form of meditation I have gone over yet, but I will do so later on in the book much more in-depth. Personal mantras allow you to bring confidence to yourself and set yourself up to finish everything you have planned for the day.
- **Energizing Breath Meditation:** This is another new form of meditation being introduced right now! However, again, I will be bringing it back up with practical exercises later on. Just now, know that energizing breath meditation allows for *Prana* to flow uninhibited through your body. It is all about release and the clearing of all channels to let energy fill you.
- **Mindfulness Meditation:** There is no better way to begin your day than with mindfulness. This will force you to put away your plans for the day and focus

primarily on bringing yourself to a point of peace. This is a great way to focus on clearing some of your chakras and meditating on them to set you up for a better path to success.

Chakras to Focus On: Root chakra, heart chakra, throat chakra

Night-time Meditation

At night, the goal is slightly different. This is your time to unwind from the day and make sure that you are letting go fully of those perceived failures you may have experienced. Many people struggle with insomnia and fatigue the next day as a result. You might be surprised to learn that this can easily by a symptom of blocked chakras. Opening up and cleansing your spiritual centers is going to let sleep come quickly, and let you rest peacefully all through the night.

- **Mindfulness Meditation:** Again, mindfulness should always be your go-to whenever you need to ready for yourself for anything. Whether it is for relaxation, spiritual enlightenment, talking in front of an audience… really, whatever! Mindfulness is the best way to bring yourself to a point where all things are possible. This is even more important at night when you need to put away all things from the day.

- **Spiritual Meditation:** Finding peace within yourself is key to getting a good night of sleep. Cleansing your chakras and letting *Prana* flow freely is key. If you are taking the spiritual route, you can easily slip in meditation with your nightly prayer routines. Even if you do not regularly pray to your deity, you can still find much to be gained. Not only are you opening up the gates to your energy, but you are also becoming closer to the God of your choosing.
- **Visualization Meditation:** While this could be used in the morning, I think it is especially potent at bringing people closer to sleep. Preferably you are going to envision yourself, sleeping peacefully, free of bad dreams or restlessness. Picturing this in your brain helps your body relax into the idea of sleep and will also set you up for a much more relaxed night.

Chakras to Focus On: Root chakra, solar plexus chakra, crown chakra

You should have a far better understanding of which time of day is best for what. Honestly, I fully recommend that you engage at both times of day for around 20 minutes each time. This will give you the full effects that you are looking for.

Once you have figured out when and where you are going to begin meditating and cleansing your chakras, it is time to move on to the next step: setting up your space. This is an important step for those who are looking to take this seriously. Any person who wants to practice Buddhism, whether as a religion or as a philosophy, needs to have the proper space in which to do so.

Making sure that this space is optimized for your experience is crucial. You cannot hope to find peace within yourself if you are not set up to do so. Of course, if you are going to begin practicing Buddhism alongside this then there are a few things you should keep in mind.

- **Stay Minimalistic:** One of the main principles of a Buddhist lifestyle is remaining minimalistic. Since the path to Nirvana is heavily involved with letting go of desire or materialism, minimalism is something Buddhists hold dear. Make sure that your space is barren of earthly possession or things you may covet. Make this space where you are surrounded by only what you need, so that you may concentrate on becoming content with just that. Only what you need, that is.

- **Focus on Sensation:** There are many ways in which to bring comfort, and heighten success without bringing in excessive materials you do not need. Incense is a popular form of bringing in a stimulating, chakra-opening presence. There are a few other ways to do this, which I will get more info below. The goal is to make sure that you are using your senses and engaging them entirely.
- **Maintain Focus:** Part of being minimalistic is bringing a clearer focus to yourself. When you are not engaged with materialistic things clogging up your area, you can begin to focus on what is important. Mindfulness will help you better cultivate your focus and help you maintain clarity while aligning your energy.
- **Further Humility:** Your main focus should always be to become more and more humble with each session. Practicing humility is not just good for Buddhists- it is good for everybody. Humility builds your resilience and creates further resistance against the stressors this world has to offer. Your life will only get better and better as you begin to further your humility through the practice of chakra cleansing and meditation.

These are all fantastic steps you can take to ensure your space is going to do what it is supposed to do: relax you through these different practices and keep you in tune with yourself and your environment.

Speaking of environment, there are a few things I suggest you always have to make sure your space is going to be up to par. While materialistic possessions are not the goal, there are a few items that will bring a certain sense of peace to you. Most Buddhists practice using:

- **Incense:** Most likely the first thing that comes to mind when you think of meditation is incense. This is one of those things that very much intertwined with Buddhist practices, as well as with Hinduism. Most eastern cultures use incense in religious tradition as a rule.

Having the right incense can make a world of a difference to clearing your chakras and reaching better alignment within yourself. There are actually different types of incense reserved for different ceremonies or reasons. However, you can generally choose the type that is most preferable to you. The goal is not to follow any pre-determined rules; it is to find your own balance and your own way through this journey.

Incense allows you to home in on a point of concentration. A large part of mindfulness is clearing your mind and focusing on the present moment. Incense gives you a better ability to do this. Nevertheless, I will talk about incense in more detail at a later stage.

- **Gong:** In some ceremonies, gongs are absolutely crucial. However, if you are looking to truly cleanse your chakras and maintain mindfulness, they are necessary all of the time. This is seen mostly in Tibetan Buddhism, however, so keep in mind that it is an offshoot.

    Ringing a gong is meant to show your affection and appreciation for the Buddha. There are also different rituals you can perform with it which are meant to bring wisdom to you and better show your compassion for the world.

- **Cushion:** Something you will become all-too-familiar within meditation is how hard the floor is. Some choose to use only a thin mat, or none whatsoever. It depends on how close to traditional practice you want to go. Buddhists believe in letting go of desire and material possession in order to move forward toward enlightenment. It is because of this that some argue cushions defeat the entire purpose as they are a luxury you do not need.

I would suggest using a cushion or mat at first in order to acclimate your body slowly to the practice. You can choose to go more minimalistic as you engage more and more with the practice.

There are different cushions used in different forms of Buddhism. In Zen Meditation, in particular, there is a Zafu. You can look into which firms require which ceremonial cushions.

- **Prayer Flags:** This is another Tibetan tradition that originated in the high Himalayan mountains. Monks originally would use them to give blessing to the world around them, but especially the countryside they called home. Prayer flags are an excellent addition to your ceremonial set-up which will bring peace by nature.
- **Wall Hangings:** Other forms of religious decoration can be found. Many wall hangings exist which are meant to remind you of your place in the world. Having wall hangings of the different chakras can also be helpful. This is especially true if you are looking to meditate on one chakra in particular. Being able to see the wall

hanging and visualize is a large part of clearing yourself and opening energy channels.
- **Buddha Statues:** This is a huge part of your shrine, should you be a practicing Buddhist. Having statues of the Buddha is not a fashion statement, or some aesthetic people choose. It is a religious practice, one deeply rooted in the practices that Buddhists take part in. Having a Buddha statue is especially important if you are looking to practice religiously. Note that this is different than having religious symbols for God. The Buddha is not a God. He is simply a man who reached true enlightenment, whose teachings we follow. Giving offerings to the Buddha is something that many Buddhists do. It is not the same as worship, however.

Placing things at the altar of your Buddha is a relinquishment of what you do not need. It is understanding that material possession is not the end goal and that you can put everything at the feet of the Buddha and live in his image.

These are all tools you can use to bring the concentration back to the meat of the matter. The goal is to build yourself in the ways that are meaningful: humility, love, peace, and more.

Create a space in which you feel most at peace and can practice these principles that will ultimately allow *Prana* to move through your body's spiritual centers uninhibited.

Chapter 4: Meditation and Chakras

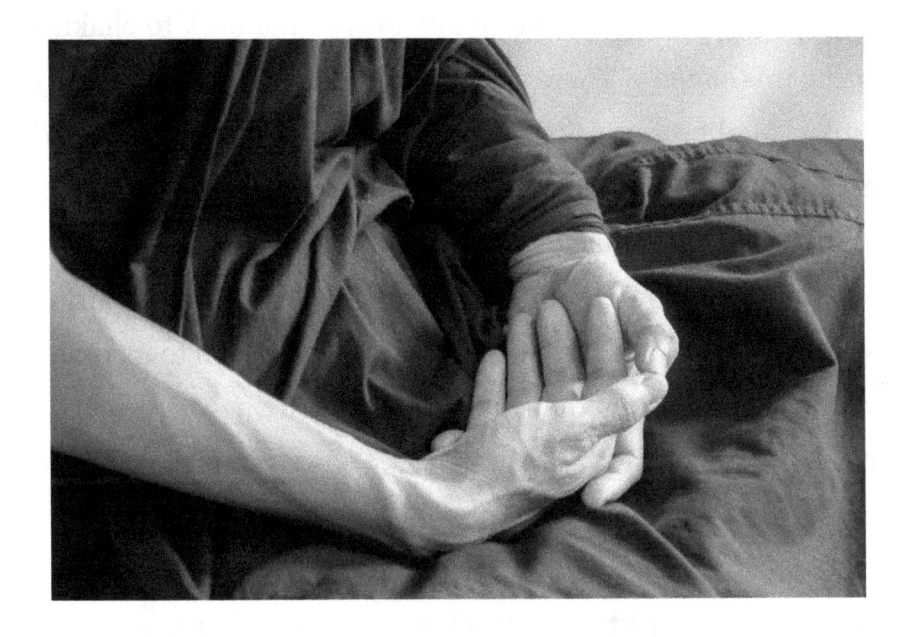

The Subtle and Not So Subtle Connection

Now that we have gone over both of these topics, at least the basics, I think I need to move into how they have connected and the different topics that start moving closer toward chakra cleansing. There is a huge difference between meditation as a whole and specific meditation-based on clearing your chakras. Many links exist and, frankly, the two terms are somewhat intertwined. However, there is enough of a difference for me to lay it out clearly for you.

First, let us talk about some of the links between chakras and meditation. I am sure you can guess what some of them are already since I made sure to relate everything back to chakras during this chapter. There are a few things which are absolutely similar. Meditation seeks to bring you back to inner peace and calm your mind. Chakras perform the same duty, though through a different means. Anybody can practice meditation. This is an open area that many wander through, or by, during their lifetime. One of the biggest reasons people fail to meditate properly, however, is that they are not enacting the powerful energy centers within themselves. Those centers being, of course, their chakras.

It is an amateur mistake to think that you can simply meditate and all of the *Prana* flowing through your body will go where it needs to. Meditation is wonderful and, as I went over earlier, has many benefits. However, you cannot hope to achieve the benefits of chakra alignment without working dutifully towards that goal. In essence, the main link is that meditation is the method through which you align your chakras. Meditation is a key element in the Buddhist tradition, alongside all other eastern philosophies.

The differences lay in the different styles of meditation that are out there. I will be going over chakra-specific meditation in the next chapter. In order for you to cleanse your chakras, you need to be very much intentional in what you do. This is an active progression that you will take further and further with each session of meditation. Chakras are not like a car. You cannot take them in to get "tuned up" once in a blue moon and feel fine. In order to access your *Prana* and free the toxins within yourself, it must be done repetitively with purpose.

As I mentioned, and showed earlier, there are several different styles of meditation out there. Not a single one is more or less useful than another. They all have a place in your life and you should be mindful about how you use them. It is a blessing that we have all of these different forms. No matter what, you know that you can access the right energy channels and the correct mind space you need at the moment.

Chakra meditation is generally speaking better than other styles because of what it offers to you. It is not just about feeling better or putting yourself on the fast track to success. In fact, many high-powered professionals who engage in meditation are missing the entire point.

Chakra meditation is vastly superior because it gets to the root of the problem and helps you find inner peace. Other forms of meditation do not have the same lasting effects. They are certainly less effective. Engaging your chakras is a huge part of making sure that you are meditating properly. It is the entire goal of meditating, in my mind. Your life energy is what determines your station in life. You cannot move forward properly and with purpose until you make sure that you are living meaningfully. Opening up your chakras allows you to do just that.

Of course, you can engage your chakras in absolutely any form of meditation. It is this, that makes them so crucial. Meditation, again, is fantastic on its own. When you begin to focus in on your chakras, however, it takes a whole new role in your life. You can include chakras in meditation through a variety of means. Sometimes people go through full-body cleanses, in which they visualize and focus on each chakra, clearing them one at a time in line.

Other times, you may find that you do not have the time to do a full-body cleanse. Or, you may have a problem in life that shows in one of your channels being blocked.

When you feel "butterflies" in your stomach, for example, this is a sign that your solar plexus chakra is particularly weak. Engaging in meditation later on when you can and focusing on that chakra, in particular, can help calm this sensation.

Even when you feel as though the sensation is positive, such as butterflies as a result of another person's affection, know that this goes against Buddhist practice. You are free to love and love you should, but it should not take over your life. Your life is not meant to be spent pouring everything into one other person. The idea of Buddhism is that we must let go of these desires- even the desire for a partner. These things will come in time as karma brings them. The road to enlightenment is undoubtedly difficult, and sometimes it is lonely. Have peace within yourself and allow life to do as it will. I am not saying in any way shape or form to leave your partner and take the lone-wolf route, but merely describing the traditional Buddhist values.

As it is, you are simply energy within a vessel. Let yourself flow.

One of the last topics I would like to go over is the idea of the subtle body. This may be something you have not heard of before, which is totally fine. It is more a niche topic related to the idea of chakras. However, it is not firmly Buddhist in nature. In fact, it is an idea that originated from Yogic people. However, you will see it used in many different ways throughout some eastern philosophies and religions.

First, I think I should explain that there are actually 3 bodies. These are the three that you will need to know about:

- **The Casual Body:** This is the innermost portion of yourself. The casual body is that which holds a veil over your soul.
- **The Subtle Body:** The body which connects the physical and the casual. This is where we experience feelings and realize sensations. It is the system through which energy moves.
- **The Physical Body:** Of course, this is the body that you reside within. Your physical body is a passing thing, and eventually, it will no longer be yours.

Each of these three play a crucial role in carrying you along your journey to enlightenment. For now, we will simply focus on the subtle body and how this relates to you. The subtle body is the connection between the physical and the casual. There are many beliefs surrounding the subtle body and, honestly, I could write an entire book just based on this alone. I will just be going over a brief history, as well as how it comes into play with Buddhism.

The subtle body is where you experience both feelings as well as sensations. It is the link between the casual body, the one which veils your soul, and the physical body, that which you reside in. The subtle body was not originally called this, and all languages have their own versions of it. However, to keep things simple, I will only be referring to it as the subtle body.

There is really no telling where the subtle body originally took hold or became a fleshed-out idea. Just as with the rest of Buddhism, and other eastern philosophies, it stretches back thousands of years. As all things do, however, it comes back to Sanskrit. It is thought that perhaps the word comes from Suksma. This is the word, which means "dormant" in Sanskrit. The word "sarira" may also come into play, which is the Sanskrit word for the body.

Many different religions understand the idea of the subtle body. Although it is most popular in eastern traditions, we also see traces of it everywhere, including the western world.

The subtle body is one that you will need to practice feeling. It is possible to have a better understanding of this realm and connecting to it comes with a host of benefits. You can better control your energy centers, which includes cleaning and opening your chakras. The subtle body is how all of these energy forms and how it connects from body to mind to soul.

Buddhists believe that the path to enlightenment is paved with an understanding of the subtle body, and your ability to impact it. Awareness is not just contained in your head or mind. In fact, awareness is a concept you need to take into consideration throughout the entirety of yourself. You cannot reach true enlightenment if you are not in touch with your subtle body and the energy, which flows through it.

Some use the subtle body as a chance to heal themselves. In fact, through breathing and other exercises, it is thought that you can fully control your subtle body. This is after much practice and movement towards enlightenment, however. Generally speaking, you want to have a teacher to lead you through these things. The subtle body is an advanced idea that will take you a long time to work through and understand.

But what is energy? And how does it relate to anything at all?

We talked about *Prana* earlier, the life force which flows through all things. However, I think we need to talk a little bit more about energy in general. Energies are something you must understand before you try and jump into advanced practice, like engaging and controlling your subtle body.

The term "energy" is simply used to mean the force that makes the world turn. It is present in all living things, and even things that are not living. Energy is present in all beings and it is the control and manipulation of these energies which brings you closer to enlightenment. The entire purpose of cleansing your chakras and opening them up is to allow that all-mighty energy to move uninhibited through you.

Energy can be manipulated. It can be used as the tool that it is. The practice of meditation, especially as it relates to Buddhists, is to do exactly this. Whether or not that is your intention, or whether or not you are even aware of it, does not matter. There is much to be said about doing these things purposefully, however, and as mentioned, the path to enlightenment calls for purpose, not a coincidence.

The idea of energies is present in every single culture dating back to the beginning of time... and even before. Many are open to the idea that there is a force in this world that we do not understand. Perhaps you have felt it during times of euphoria, or moments of complete peace. These are all events that can spark a more harmonious relationship with the subtle body. We all feel it, and we all know it exists regardless of conscious understanding. It dictates much about us. The subtle body and chakras are entirely complementary in nature.
Our bodies are made up of flesh, blood, and bone, yes. But they are also made up of sheets of vibrating energy. Each one of these layers has a purpose in the grand scheme of things, and each is important to your happiness and health. The fact of the matter is that our physical body is but a vessel full of energy. Part of maintaining a path to enlightenment is understanding the impermanence of the physical body, and doing your due diligence to ensure oneness with the subtle body.

The subtle body is the system through which chakras connect. Chakras are simply points of energy within this subtle body. It is the flow of energy through these vibrating layers in every system of self. Your subtle body suffers when your chakras are blocked due to the lack of *Prana*. Your chakras can be thought of as gateways that your energy passes through.

In order to maximize your wellbeing and bring you to a state of completion, you must focus on your connection to your subtle body. This is where the true power in cleansing your chakras lay. You will never be able to expand your consciousness into the subtle body if you are not able to clear your chakras properly. On that note, it is time to move into the next chapter. In this coming chapter, I am finally going to get into the world of chakra meditation! We are now ready to begin learning the secrets to keeping chakras clear and becoming more in tune with ourselves as a result. I am very excited to move with you through this next section, which will go over all of the exercises you need to formulate your plan for wellness.

Chapter 5: Chakra Meditation for Beginners

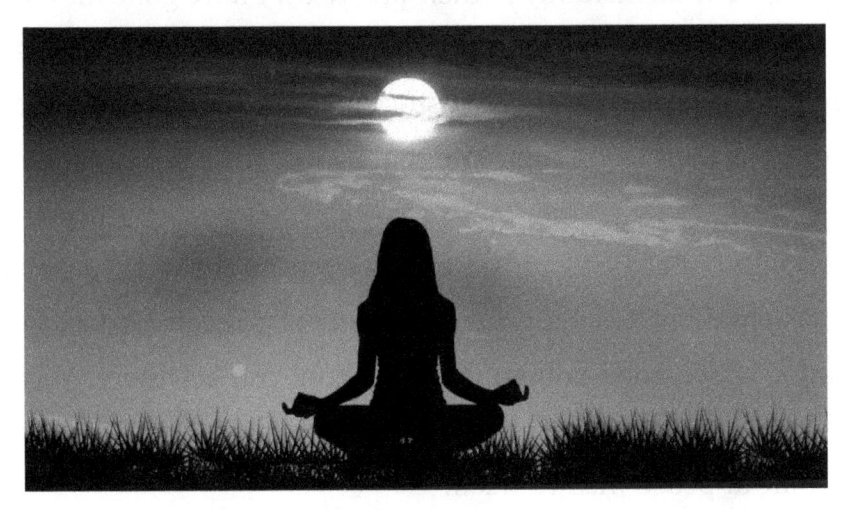

All Things Related to the Basis of this Book

We went over chakra meditation briefly in the previous chapter. This entire chapter, however, will be dedicated to exactly that. Remember when I promised to give you some helpful exercises and practical meditation guides? This is the chapter in which I am going to give you all of that information… and more!

First, I would like to talk a little bit more about the history of charka meditation specifically, and the different branches, which use it consistently in their practices. I have gone into the history of other topics, and I do not want to bore you. Because of this, I will make sure the history is brief. I know you are as excited as I am to get right into the thick of things!

Clearing your chakras and becoming one with the world around you is possible. Reaching enlightenment is possible. It does not matter which road you go down or how you get there. What matters is that your energy is flowing freely, and you have become at peace with yourself.

Aligning your energy is the part at which both Tantric Buddhism and all other forms of this practice meet. The energy that makes the world around us work, the *Prana*, is the ultimate goal we are trying to understand. Just because you do not want to practice religiously does not mean there are not avenues you can go down. Clearing out your chakras is not releasing your faith. In fact, the only things you are releasing are your negative thought patterns and your lack of connection to the world around you.

Healing your spirit is the goal of all of these different philosophies and religions. The point I am trying to make is that, at the end of the day, almost all religions come back to this idea. We all recognize the energy within us, although we have called it different names. Some may refer to its entirety as a "soul", while others may use the term "spirit". The most ancient of religions, however, know it to simply be energy.

It is only through the correction of energy flow that we can achieve true healing of the spirit. You can feel your chakras are blocked through every part of your body. Each of these has its own role to play, which I will go over exclusively in the next chapter. There is a long list of ailments which are caused by a blockage of any chakra, even those which are going to go unnamed for this book. Remember: we do not have only the 7 chakras. There are many other systems that utilizes other amounts, such as the 12 chakra system. The seven chakra system is one of the most know and beginner-friendly. These are merely the gateways for energy, and so we have many all over our bodies. If you remember from earlier, I stated that there are approximately 114.

This high number makes sense and is highly intuitive to the idea of spirit, soul, or energy. We recognize that it flows through our entirety. Buddhism and the idea of chakras simply put it in more physical, tangible terms. It is funny since often "new age" beliefs are considered "whacky" or "out there". The fact of the matter is that the religions which formed later pulled from these ancient traditions. Believing in chakras is not believing in magic. We have known since the beginning of ourselves that chakras exist. This is why so many have spoken of it, even in different ways, throughout our history.

Every major religion or philosophy generally has some component of life energy or force within it. Chakras are just the gateways through which that force passes and travels.

In order to ensure that you are in full connection with yourself, I am now going to talk about how, exactly, to do that. I think the chapters which prelude this one did a wonderful job of explaining why chakras are so important. Aligning your energy is not just about a spiritual connection. It is that, yes, but it is so much more. Aligning your energy is about ensuring that your physical body is primed and taken care of. All things fall into line when you can ensure that you are soaking up as much as *Prana* as you need to.

When any part of our chakras is clouded we feel the effects in numerous ways. Fatigue, loneliness, anxiety, anger; negative emotions of every shape and size are brought to light when we neglect this most basic part of ourselves.

If you are familiar with Maslow's hierarchy, let me draw a more modern way in which we understand the idea of chakras. This is a triangle that leads from physiological needs to the idea of "self-actualization". Maslow is simply drawing from an idea that the Buddha himself drew up. The base of the triangle is the first step in becoming the best version of you. It is comprised of necessities for example food, shelter, and other such things.

You can think of this as your body. This is the first area you must care for if you wish to truly achieve an enlightened state. From here, the triangle builds upwards until it reaches the peak. It goes through different levels of things you must have before you can reach the pinnacle. In the case of Maslow's Hierarchy, this is called self-actualization. In the case of the Path to Enlightenment, it is called Nirvana.

Many philosophers who are now widely famous can credit their thought patterns to Buddhist tradition. You will find more and more that the idea of chakras simply makes sense. You will also find more and more that as you clear your chakras and care for them, your journey through life will become easier.

The negative effects of untended chakras range in both variety and severity. You will find in most cases, however, that these effects are easily managed when you reach the right meditative state.

Speaking of meditative states, I think it is time to teach you how to unblock your chakras. First, however, I will go over everything you need to know to be set up for success. Below I will list out breathing techniques you will use in order to increase energy flow, calm your mind, and make mindfulness come easily.

Breathing Exercises

The first step in this process is ensuring that you know how to breathe correctly. There is much that goes into breathing and, unfortunately, most of the practice lazy breathing which, in of itself, can cause our chakras to cloud over. We must invite energy in with our inhale and let out the negative on the exhale. I will take you through quite a few and tell you how to complete them. We will not quite get into the practice of clearing chakras yet. There is a certain amount of set-up required for you to be effective.

Essentially, I am teaching this to you in the same order that a teacher or educator on the topic would. The same way I was taught. I think that makes the most sense, after all! I will also include a few simple exercises which can be used anywhere. I think this is important because it helps you have better tend to your blocked chakras or problems with *Prana* flow anywhere. Chakras require near-constant attention. However, as you become more aware of them, it will come easily to you to do so daily.

- **Roaring Breath:** This practice is a great way to engage your throat chakra. First, sit cross-legged. Raise upward through your crown chakra, feeling yourself pushing upward. Breathe in deeply, engaging your diaphragm entirely. You will then exhale with an entirely open mouth. As you do so, growl low in your throat. Yes, like a Lion. Make sure you are keeping your breath even as you both inhale and exhale.

- **Alternating Nostrils:** A very simplistic exercise, this is one that I highly recommend you begin incorporating into your day. This will help you build up to exercises that require a little more "stamina" in your lungs. At first, practicing "proper breathing" can make you dizzy. This is because you are not used to the oxygen intake.

To begin using this, you will bring yourself to a state of clear mindfulness, as always. You will do this for all the exercises. This will bring you into a state of being more focused and alert and is best done before going into a meeting or some other important event. Breathing using this technique is fairly involved. This is why it works to make you more alert. First, using your right hand, you will bend your pointer and middle finger so that they are laying on the palm of your hand. From here, you will bring your hand up to your face. Using the thumb of this hand, close your nostrils to the right. Inhale through the left, and then slide it over to the other side and repeat. You will move back and forth between your two nostrils.

- **Bellowing Breath:** If you are feeling uptight and anxious, this is a great exercise to perform. It can also be highly energizing in the morning so you can feel awakened and ready for your day. Feeling the afternoon slump? This is your answer! However, keep in mind that it does look a little bit ridiculous.

  Most things which work so well tend to!

  You can do this one sitting or standing up. First, you are going to take your hands and form them into fists. Raise them above your head, keeping them straight and relaxed. If it feels good, feel free to stretch a little upward, too.

  This is a great breathing exercise to use for engaging Crown chakra and focusing the *Prana* through your body. Let out a loud exhale, saying the word "AH!" as you do. The idea is to release stress and push out the negative thoughts that plague you. Focus on how the breath feels leaving you, and the goodness you bring in when you inhale. Swing your arms down to your sides, as well, on the exhale. You can also punch the air if that feels better.
- **Kapalabhati Breathing:** A mind-clearing exercise, this form of breathing is specifically about cleansing your chakras and increasing your energy. It is meant to bring balance to your body and *Prana*. It also is fantastic

for getting your blood flowing. Begin in a sitting position, preferably in the same position you meditate in.

You will first put your hands together in front of you, with your fingertips facing upward. After this, pull in the air gently, all the way into your stomach. Then, blow out through your nose. You want to bounce your naval up and down. This is a great exercise for engaging your sacral and solar plexus chakras.

- **3-Part Breathing:** The goal of this exercise is to bring you into a state of calm. It is best performed before bed so that you can have sounder sleep and fall asleep more quickly. It helps restore you and is great for aligning chakras and getting your *Prana* flowing freely.

You will place your hands on the heart chakra and the sacral chakra. Instead of engaging in diaphragm breathing, you will pull air right into your chest cavity. After this, puff out your belly while holding the breath. Now, exhale slowly. Repeat this process with slow and even breathing.

- **Ocean Breath:** Thought to be the most commonly used technique, there is Ocean Breath. This is also referred, more technically, as Ujjayi breath. It is easy to use and can be used alongside many different activities and in any situation. Note that I consider this an "advanced" exercise. This is because it involves breathing that might make you dizzy. You need to start with simpler exercises to get your body used to the large quantities of oxygen you are bringing into your body.

In order to do Ocean Breath, you are going to sit in a comfortable position, preferably in the same one you meditate in.
Now, breathe in deeply, and slowly, through your nose. When you breathe in, engage "throat breathing". This is when you open your throat and pull in the air with it. You should hear a slight "hiss" as you do so. Some people compare it to the sound of the ocean! This is where the name comes from.
Exhale slowly, making sure to keep it even with the inhale. You will simply repeat this for approximately five minutes.

Mindfulness Exercises

Cultivating a constant state of mindfulness is not out of your reach. There are many people who are able to practice it daily and begin to implement it in their daily lives. Mindfulness is a form of meditation that can help you clear your chakras. Because of this, I am going to go over all of the different ways you can do this.

Note that you can turn any of these into a chakra cleansing exercise. I will get more into clearing your chakras later, but for now, know that all exercises provided can be taken a step further in that way. That is why I am giving you this foundation!

- **Yawn and Stretch:** Believe it or not, this simple task is not only great for your body, but it is also great for practicing mindfulness. Getting up and moving around often is great for your body. This is especially true if you are working at a desk or sitting down all day. You simply clear your mind entirely and focus only on how your body feels. Do not think about words such as "tightness" or "sore". Instead, simply pinpoint and be generally aware of that ache or pain.

    Once you have pinpointed it, just gently stretch. You can swing your body around slowly, bend over and slowly touch your toes... anything you want! Just do what feels good and gets your body loose. Make sure you are only focusing on the feelings and sensations at this time. This is also a great exercise to get more in touch with the subtle body. It helps your physical body connect with that undercurrent of vibration.

- **Hand Massaging:** Another simple exercise, this is something you can do practically anywhere. If you type a lot then this is going to be something you should engage with often. Simply take your hands and begin rubbing the tendons gently. Stretch out your fingers by bending them slowly backward. Massage the joints and your knuckles. Experiment with you stretches and do what feels good to you.

During this, focus on the sensation of massaging your hands. Close your eyes and home in on that warm, relaxing feeling. Recognize how your skin feels under your fingers and the warmth of your hands. Keep your mind clear and live in this pleasant experience. It also feels really great, especially once you begin doing it regularly.

- **Body Scan:** Especially useful for those who live with chronic pain, body scans keep you in tune with your physical body. This is another great way to begin getting in touch with the subtle body and bringing it to your attention. You will simply find somewhere to sit or, more preferably, lay down. If you are sitting, place your palms facing upwards on your thighs. If laying down, lay your arms beside you, also with palms facing up.

Relax your entire body. You will begin at the crown chakra. Tense your head and hold this for three seconds or so. Release entirely, and slowly, feeling the tension slowly fade. Move down to the throat chakra and tense again. And, once more, release. You will repeat this all the way down, focusing on tensing your body one section at a time focusing on the Prana gateways. Once you have done this a couple of times, you should be able to more readily release tension through your entire body. After getting to this point, you will begin the actual body scan. Focus on one point of your body at a time, clearing your mind and thinking only in terms of sensation. You are activating the connection with your subtle body during this exercise.

Try and look for aches and pains. Once you have identified them, you will know where you need to stretch and which parts you need to better take care of.

- **Positive Mantras:** One of my favorite ways to begin the day is with positive mantras. The form of mindfulness can bring such positive energy into your life and bring your energy into balance in so many ways. There is something to be said about cultivating a positive mindset and putting it to use daily. You will see your confidence rise, calmness reflected in your daily life, and a newfound desire to move forward through life.

In order to practice this, you first need to figure out which things you are moving toward. Releasing your desires does not mean giving up on life. You still should move forward, but with kindness and humility. Do what you are drawn to, and what you think will be the biggest contribution towards the world that you can muster. Do no harm but do as much as you can.

Bring to mind affirming, positive things. These can be simple words or short sentences. Whatever inspires you and brings you a feeling of calm. You will close your eyes, sitting down, and begin clearing your mind. If you want, you can start with a body scan. Once you are in a state of mindfulness, which is the absence of concrete thought, begin to slowly chant those words or phrases through your mind. Focus on each word, using your inner voice to say them confidently, but mentally.

Be firm with yourself but also be gentle. You must learn to be patient and know that if you follow the Four Noble Truths, you will be well on your way to positive events. After all, that is how karma works. You should always be moving towards accumulating good karma!

- **Visualization:** The last exercise I will go over is visualization. When you are attempting to manifest good things and pull them toward you, the best thing to do is cultivate your kindness and lower your ego. Some methods of visualization encourage you to imagine big, fancy houses and other materialistic endeavors you may be undertaking. However, this is a much different way to do this.

I recommend thinking about ways in which you can help the world. Bring yourself to a point of mindfulness, sitting in a comfortable position. Clear your mind, breathe evenly, and begin to allow your mind to form images. Some people have problems envisioning things in their brains, so for those of you, I recommend sticking to positive mantras with the same idea behind them.

Begin to think about the positive impact you can have and imagine yourself doing these things. This is the first step in pulling the opportunity toward you in order to help others. Also, visualize success, but as it relates to non-materialistic things. If you are arguing with a friend, imagine how you two will make up and what that exchange will look like. Will these problems to unravel and solve.

I hope that helps you as you begin to prepare for doing exercises more in tune with *Prana* and the flow of it through the spiritual gateways in your body. You can practice most of them in your day-to-day life as you go about your activities. I would recommend taking some time and doing so. It is an amazing advantage to have for all the benefits, which come with it.

Now that we have gone over different exercises, I want to go more in-depth on setting up your space. I am going to go over a few different types of incense, and other ideas for furthering your spiritual connection to the subtle body. Having the correct place to practice is half of the battle. You need to make sure you are ready and practicing your form of chakra meditation while honoring the idea of Buddhist philosophies. I want to make sure you understand how best to set up the space for spiritual growth. I will do so in order so that you know where to start, and everything else right down to the last step.

Finding the Right Space

There is something special about being set up in a space meant just for meditation. This is the best way to tackle it as you can easily make your space entirely customized to your spiritual needs. Clearing your chakras and enabling *Prana* to flow is not about setting, perhaps, but the setting certainly does help.

You can also use other things in this space in order to help you achieve your meditative goals. I will go over those after this. For now, here are some great places where you can set up your area:

- **Your Room:** One of the most popular places to have space is in the bedroom. This gives you the ability to easily wake up and go to sleep engaging in meditation and tending to your chakras. However, you may want to steer clear of this if you struggle with insomnia. While meditation and making sure your gateways are open, it is fantastic for trouble sleeping. However, associating anything besides sleep with the bedroom can be a problem for your brain. Those with insomnia should avoid doing anything but sleeping in their bedrooms.
- **Office Space:** If you are lucky enough to have an office at home, using it for this dual-purpose is going to be a fantastic idea. Not only will you make this space more friendly for spiritual growth and mindfulness, but you will also be able to stop and practice during the day. Most will find the largest benefits from consistent tending during their waking hours.
- **Backyard:** Nature is a focal point for many looking to find their connection to the world around us. A backyard is a wonderful place to practice meditating and getting your chakras ready to accept and release your energies. If you do not have a private space in your backyard,

however, you may want to skip this idea. It can be difficult to practice when you are out in the open and feeling weird about others seeing you.

Closet space: Finally, this is actually my favorite method. Closets are small, confined spaces that you can control the lighting of completely. Most like to meditate in a fairly dim place. This helps you relax and get into the correct mindset. You do not need much space and can easily set up a small shrine as well as a couple of wall hangings even in a smaller closet. Give it a try! You may be surprised at how much you like it.

I also think it is perfectly in line with the idea of minimalism and humility. This space is not extravagant or large. It is a reminder of your small part in the world and the peace you must make with the release of the physical body's desires.

Types of Incense

This may seem like a strange thing to bring up. However, incense is a huge part of a practicing Buddhist's life. Even when you are only following the philosophy, it is still a powerful ceremonial tool to help you. There is much more to incense than you may think. I will go over the two main types below and in what situations you should use them.

- **Stick:** This is what you normally think of when you think about incense. There are two different types. One is filled with bamboo and does not burn completely because of this. The other is coreless stick incense. This type burns away completely into ash. For this reason, it is mostly preferred for ceremonial or Buddhist purposes.

You can also offer stick incense to the Buddha. This is a wonderful show of affection for this enlightened man. When you do this you should bow in front of your shrine, palms together and pointing toward the Buddha statue. You will light the incense from this position, leaving one hand in the same position but flipping the other forward to light the incense.

When you put it out, if you cannot allow it to burn entirely out, do not blow on it. This is considered highly disrespectful. In some cultures, it is akin to spitting on the incense. Instead, to practice in true Buddhist style, hold it burning tip up, and pull down quickly. You can also use your hand to wave the flame out.

- **Loose:** While a more traditional method of practicing, this is normally only found in temples at this point. This incense can be tricky because it requires burning coal in order to use. You can actually buy hot coals, however, at any store, which sells Hookah supplies. If you would like to go this route, light the coal and let it get nice and hot.

From here, you will take a pinch of the incense between your fingers. You are going to raise this to your forehead briefly, and then sprinkle it onto the coil.

Types of Candles

While it may seem like a small detail, candles are an incredibly important part of practicing Buddhism and clearing chakras. There are some, which are specifically for ceremonial use or designed as offering to the Buddha. You do not need to spend extravagant money, however, on these candles. Indeed, it may be better to carefully carve symbols into the candles yourself. The entire idea of Buddhism is to let go of material possession and other desires, after all.

- **Container Candles:** These are candles that burn in the container you buy them in. They are fine to use, but it is preferable to use candles that go into a container you have. You can choose ceremonial candleholders specifically designed for Buddhist practice. You want them to be minimal and humble in nature.
- **Pillar Candles:** Those thick, large candles are pillar candles. They are fantastic for use with Buddhist or

meditative practices. You can even buy some, which are engraved with chakra symbols.

- **LED Fake Tealights:** For those of you who are not able to burn candles, using fake tealights is a great option. There is no danger in leaving them on, after all. I recommend this to those who may be particularly forgetful. This does not diminish your offering.
- **Tapering Candles:** This type of candle is used quite a bit at restaurants. It is the long, slender, slightly tapering style. They are fantastic for Buddha statues, which are larger. I think that using a candle that is around the same size makes a better, more thoughtful offering.

This is where I will be leaving you on this topic! In the next chapter, we are going to dive right into an explanation of all of your chakras. You can consider chapter four as your chakra field guide. Anytime you need information on a chakra, just flip it open and find what you need to know easily!

Chapter 8: Closing Thoughts for You

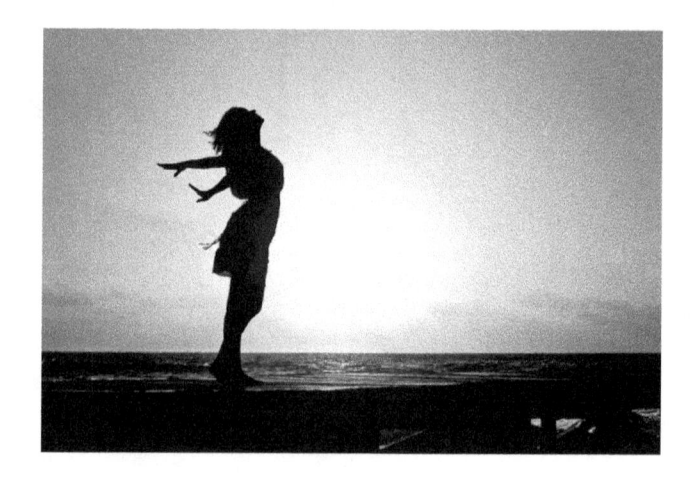

Some Thoughts to Clarify and Further Enlighten

We have finally come to the last chapter in this book! I am going to leave you with some ideas about the differences in yoga and chakra meditation. I will also go over Kundalini yoga, which is the practice of awakening your dormant energy. This last chapter will encompass many topics that will tie everything together, I promise. Thank you for reading this far, and I hope this last chapter fills you in on everything else you need to know.

There is a difference between yoga and chakra meditation. One of these is an overarching practice with a rich history in multiple different parts of Eastern philosophy.

The other is a very specific type of cleansing ritual that is meant to help your *Prana* flow freely. You can incorporate the two together and obtain some amazing results for yourself. This is why I separated those topics out a little bit so that you would have a better idea of how they disconnect, and where, exactly, they do connect.

One specific branch of yoga, Kundalini yoga, is meant expressly to help you awaken dormant energy. It is actually a combination of different practices, both Raja, Bhakti and Shakti yoga.

- **Raja Yoga:** A practice aimed towards gaining better control of yourself through both meditative and physical approaches.
- **Bhakti Yoga:** A branch of yoga that focuses on chanting and other devotions.
- **Shakti Yoga:** A style of yoga that helps you better express your energy.

These three come together in perfect harmony to form Kundalini yoga. The entire idea of this practice is to awaken that dormant energy within you, which is normally seen as a "snake" in your spine. When you are struggling with dormant energy, that snake will be coiled tightly at the base, right near your root chakra. It is your job to use Kundalini yoga in order to encourage this "snake" to uncoil and work its way up to your spine towards your crown chakra.

Kundalini actually comes from the Sanskrit word for "circular", which is "kundal".

There are a few differences between chakra meditation and Kundalini yoga. Here are a few of them:

- Kundalini yoga focuses on dormant energy, whereas chakra meditation works with the chakras themselves.
- Chakra meditation encompasses many different types of yoga.
- Kundalini is entirely its own "thing".

These are the simplest ways to tell them apart. It can be difficult to understand once you begin getting into all of these different types of yoga and meditation. That is why I saved it for last!

There are two ways in which a Kundalini class will start. These two steps are necessary to do, even if you are just trying to practice it at home.

- **Tuning In:** Making sure that you are in tune with yourself, and the world around you, is a huge first step for Kundalini yoga. You will begin each session with chanting a positive mantra. This is meant to bring neutrality to your mind and clear yourself of all doubt or bias.

You will bring your hands to your heart chakra, flat with palms together and fingertips pointing up. Chant this softly, increasing with volume as you feel your energy uncoil and your chakras awaken. Allow yourself to fall into mindfulness and practice your breathing.

- **Bowing to Your Truth:** There is a specific mudra that is associated with this process. You are going to use this mantra once you have fallen into a state of meditative fulfillment. It is the following:

"Ong Namo Guru Dev Namo"

This translates to "bowing to the truth within you".

Once you have done both of these two steps, you can begin to practice Kundalini yoga. This is a specific branch that has many different poses, mantras, and mudras. The best way to get involved in, again, to go to a class where a spiritual guide will help you through the different phases. Kundalini yoga is especially important to have a guide for because of how advanced it is. You need to make sure your chakras are aligned, clear, and strong. That is the basis of having a successful Kundalini session.

That is what you need to know about Kundalini yoga for now. I am going to now give you some tips and tricks to take with you on your journey to becoming a Yogi. This is most likely the direction you will go in if you truly want to align your chakras and become enlightened to the Four Noble Truths of the world.

Tips for Aspiring Yogis

- **Go at your own pace.** Do not let others set this for you. It is important to take this journey as you need to. There is a lot to clearing your chakras and becoming in tune with your *Prana*. When you begin to practice yoga, there are a lot of poses, too, which will be challenging. Listen to your body, both the physical and subtle, and make sure you do not take on too much at once.

- **Begin with meditation and breathing.** In the same vein, I want to remind you that you should always use this book in the right order. That is the reason I presented everything I did in the order, which I did. Begin with the first exercises I gave to you, and slowly move your way into the more advanced techniques. This is going to help you cultivate stronger energy and a better connection with the *Prana* both within you, and in the world around you.
- **Decide how you are going to tackle this.** As I mentioned, you do not need to practice Buddhism in order to activate and cleanse your chakras. However, you will find that the title will fit whether you want it or not. All of it is intrinsically connected. You will need to decide whether you wish to practice Buddhism actively, or perhaps only take the tenants you like. I always recommend it as a philosophy to stick to. This allows you to keep your current faith while still expanding your horizons.
- **Find a fantastic spiritual guide to help you.** Normally you can find somebody at a yoga studio. I recommend that you take a class, perhaps once a week, in order to better start your journey. There is much I can tell you (I already have!), but to be truly successful you

should always have somebody more knowledgeable at hand. This will help you do these meditation exercises correctly and give you a better understanding of the topics at hand.

I hope that these tips were useful... and that the rest of the book was, too! I think you will find that your life will change for the better once you are able to bring your chakras back into balance. This is all information meant to help you live a longer, healthier life, and become entirely at peace. The path to enlightenment is hard and long. That is the entire point, however. Life is not meant to be easy. In fact, that first Truth we spoke about says exactly that. Existence is suffering! We have the knowledge and tools to move away from this suffering, however, by following the eightfold path.

No matter how you choose to practice, I hope that you are able to cultivate the empathy, inner peace, and love that caring for your chakras offers.

Conclusion

Thank you for making it through to the end of *Chakra Meditation*, I hope it was informative and able to provide you with all of the tools you need to achieve your goals whatever they may be.

The next step is to begin putting into play your newfound knowledge. I have guided you through a spiritual journey and provided you with many reasons to learn more about chakras. This beginner's guide was meant to be your way of dipping your toes into the world of Buddhism, meditation, mindfulness, chakras, and how they all relate.

I hope that you have a much better understanding of what, exactly, is necessary to begin your daily rituals. As mentioned, there are things that you should always consider doing when you are beginning to put together your space. I want you to remember that first and foremost you need to be comfortable where you practice. Releasing your energy and allowing it to flow freely should be a marriage of yourself to the world around you. In order to achieve the perfect Zen, make sure you are in the perfect setting.

There is far more to open up your chakras than that, of course, but you are aware of that at this point.

The guided meditations and other exercises I put into this book were designed to get you more motivated to begin practicing these life-altering, mind-freeing routines. I promise you that your spirit and inner peace will blossom with each and every measured breath you take. From your crown to your root, everything will fall into place.

While medication is necessary in some cases, it is proven that engaging in spiritual exercises and mind-clearing activity is fantastic for mental illness. In fact, there are some solid scientific studies to back this up. I know that in the realm of spiritualism science is not always up for discussion. There is this strange misunderstanding that you have to believe in one or the other.

This could not be further from the truth!

One of the reasons meditation and mindfulness are taking the world by storm is because it works. Both are used in a large number of therapies and social-emotional learning environments. Once people become involved with these practices, they are cleaning and caring for their chakras without even knowing.

The reason you picked up this book, however, is because you want to know more about the magic behind these wonderful tools bestowed upon us by the force of the world around us. I hope that at this point you have all the tools you need for this endeavor! Enjoy your new-found knowledge and put it to use. Your body, mind, and spirit will thank you.

If you would like to know more about Chakras, check out my other books on the topic.

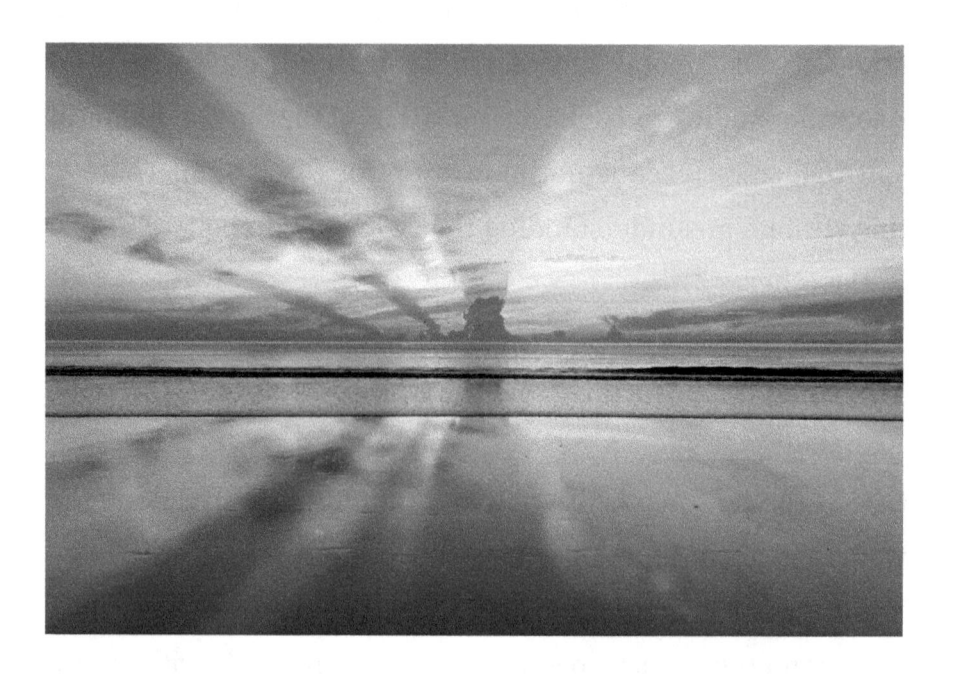

CPSIA information can be obtained
at www.ICGtesting.com
Printed in the USA
BVHW070002100321
602113BV00012B/1078